# LIVING

# A

# HAPPY LONG

# LIFE

# ON EARTH

ISBN: 9781730942808

Ben Williams

- SUPPORT YOUR BODY ABILITY TO HEAL BY EATING ENOUGH PROTEIN.

- KEEP YOUR VATALITRY ENJOYING A DIET WITH DIVERSE FRUIT AND VEGETABLE.

- EAT HEALTHY AMOUT OF CARBOHYDRATE.

- EAT A CONTROLL AMOUT OF FAT

- EAT ENOUGH VITAMINE AND MINERIALS THROUGH A HEALTHY DIET.

- EAT A LOW SALT DIET.

- CLEANSE YOUR BODY BY DRINKING ENOUGH WATER

## CHAPTER THREE.

## REDUCING STRESS

- PROTECT YOUR PSYCHOLOGICAL WELL BEING BY MAINTAING CLOSE SOCIAL RELATIONSHIP.

- STAY RESILLENT BY SLEEPING ENOUGH .

- STAY EXCITED ABOUT LIFE THROUGH HOBBIES.

- RESEARCH ILLNESSES

- CONSIDER BECOMING VEGAN OR VEGETARIAN.

# PREFACE

There are many uncertainties in life, and no one can predict how long they will live. However, there are some measures that research have proven to be the secret of living a desirable years on earth which will be discuss in this book.

## INTRODUCTION

There are many uncertainties in life which no one can predict how long and healthy they will live. However, taking good care of yourself  help to support and increase your chances of living a longer life. Take good care of your physical and psychological health by living a healthy lifestyle, eat balance diet and put your stress under control.

**get your body ready for a long life by exercising.**

 Exercise benefits both your physical and  psychological health. Physical activity strengthens your body system and helps you to put your weight under control, and also improves your balance and coordination.
Simultaneously, your body give out  endorphins which will help you feel relax and feel good. Endorphins can also reduce pain and give you good mood.

Try to  both aerobic exercise and strength training.

Aerobic exercise put your heart rate up and improves your endurance training. Possible activities that can assist you include jogging, fast walking, swimming, etc. Try to do 75 to 150 minutes every week.

Strength training, like weight lifting, improves your bone density and help to build your muscle. Try to do it two times in a  week.

**Be proactive about identifying and treating health problems.**

Preventative measures is important for identifying health problems before they become a major concern. It is also important to choose a  lifestyle factors, familial history, and work exposures that may likely lead to the development of a disease or dysfunction. If you miss a doctor's appointments, you increase the chances of not catching a developing health problem right at the beginning. This means that it will likely be more complicated and difficult to treat.

Have a checkup once in every year. If your doctor recommends other screenings, do them.

If you have a chronic health condition, talk to your doctor about how to manage it to either improve it or prevent it from getting worse.

Know what health problems may run in your family and go for appointment regularly.

**Avoid high risk behavior.**

 Accidents, including during sports or while driving, are major causes of head trauma and spinal cord injuries.

Always Drive carefully, always put on your seat belt, and obey speed limits.

Apply caution when crossing the street as a pedestrian. Watch  both ways carefully to see if there are any vehicle coming.

Always Wear the recommended  protective and safety gear when playing sports, particularly risky sports like football, horseback riding, rock climbing, bungee jumping, skydiving, skiing, and snowboarding

## Avoid toxic substances.

It is important to avoid substances that may double up your chances of developing health problems. This includes pollutants materials, pesticides materials, chemical fumes materials, and asbestos materials.

## Avoid excessive alcohol intake.

If you do drink, daily recommendations are that women should stop drinking  more than one drink in a day day and men no more than one or two drinks in a day day.

Drinking alcohol in lower quantities should be ok for your health as long as you are healthy and don't abuse it.

Excessive drinking can make you more likely to develop cancers of the digestive tract, heart problems, strokes, high blood pressure, liver disease, and to suffer injuries in accidents.[5]

If you do drink, be mindful not to mix alcohol with medicines, including over-the-counter medicines, that may interact.

Don't drink and drive

**Stop smoking and taking  nicotine products.**

 Even if you're addicted to smoking or used other nicotine products for many years, quitting will still improve your health quality  and help you live and enjoy longer life. Smoking does more harm than good to the body system. smoking greatly increases your risks of the following:

Lung diseases, including cancer

Cancer of the gullet, larynx, throat, mouth, bladder, pancreas, kidney, and cervix

Heart diseases

Strokes and high blood pressure

Diabetes

Eye problem like cataracts

Respiratory problem

 Teeth Gum disease

**Avoid street drugs.**

Street drugs are dangerous for some reasons.the drugs may not only harm you  it may also be mixed with other harmful substances. The health risks include:

Dehydration

Confusion

Memory loss

Psychosis

Seizures

Coma

Brain damage

Death

CHAPTER TWO

EATING A HEALTHY DIET.


**Support your body's ability to heal by eating enough protein.**

Your body make  use of protein to produce  new cells. This implies that it is important for repairing tissue damage in your body.

Though meat and animal are common sources of

13

protein, you can as well get all of the proteins you need from plant foods, such as lentils, beans, hemp seeds, quinoa, chia seeds, seeds, and nuts.

Proteins are present in meat, milk, fish, eggs, soy, beans, legumes, and nuts.

Adults should eat 2 to 3 servings of high protein foods in a day. Children' needs will differ according to their ages.

**Keep your vitality by enjoying a diet with diverse fruits and vegetables.**

Fruits are foods that come from the flower of plants while vegetables are foods that come from the stems, flower buds leaves, and roots. Both are very good sources of the vitamins and minerals your body require to live healthy throughout a long life.

Fruits are berries, beans, corn, peas, cucumber, grains, nuts, olives, peppers, pumpkin, squash, sunflower seeds, and tomatoes. while Vegetables include celery, lettuce, spinach, cauliflower, broccoli, beets, carrots, and potatoes.

Fruits and vegetables are low sources of calories and fat, but high in fiber and vitamins. Eating a diet of a high proportion of  fruits and vegetables can reduce your risks of developing cancer, heart diseases, high blood pressure, strokes, and diabetes.

always eat 4 servings of fruits and 5 servings of vegetables in a  day.

## **Eat healthy amounts of carbohydrates.**

 Carbohydrates are surplus in nature, such as in fruits and vegetables. Which include sugars, starches, and fiber your body generate energy by breaking down these compounds. Simple sugars are digested more easily than complex sugars.

Learn to always get most of your carbohydrates from natural sources like fruits and vegetables and cut down your intake of carbohydrates from items like baked

15

goods and other processed foods.

Simple sugars are gotten from fruits, milk, milk products, vegetables, and processed sweets.

Complex carbohydrates found in beans, peas, lentils, peanuts, potatoes, corn, green peas, parsnips, whole-grain breads.

 half of your daily calories are suppose  to  come from carbohydrates, with most of it coming from complex carbohydrates as opposed to simple sugars.

**Eat a controlled amount of fat.**

Your body needs some amount fat to help it absorb fat soluble vitamins, control inflammation, help  with muscle repair, clot blood and maintain proper and reliable brain function, but too much is not good.

Commonly sources that fat are gotten are butter, cheese, whole milk, cream, meats, and vegetable oils.

Eating high amount of fat increases your chances of high

cholesterol, heart problems, and strokes. You can reduce  the amount of  fat consumption by eating lean meats, poultry, fish, and drinking low-fat milk.

Many restaurants support  the flavor of their foods with ingredients that have  high amount of  fat such as cream, whole milk, or butter. By cooking your food yourself, you can control the amount of fat in your food.

Don't choose foods that are fat completely free. You need fat. on Contrary to popular beliefs, dietary fat does not make you fat. However, don't consume too much fat as it is unhealthy and unsafe for you.

**Eat enough vitamins and minerals through a healthy diet.**

 When your diet is balanced, you are probably getting sufficient vitamins and minerals. These substances are important for your body to function properly, repair itself and grow.

Vitamins and minerals are found  naturally in many foods, especially fruits, vegetables, whole grains, meats, and dairy.

If you are concerned that you may not be getting enough vitamins and minerals, see your doctor about adding some multivitamin and multi-mineral supplements to your diet.

The needs of pregnant women and children differ from one person to another.

## Eat a low salt diet.

While your body needs some salt too so that you can maintain muscle and nerve function and manage your blood volume and pressure and blood volume, too much over a long period of time is very unhealthy. The CDC recommends keeping your sodium consumption below 2,300 milligrams in a day.

Too much salt can cause high blood pressure and escalate heart, liver, or kidney problems.

Most foods contain some salt naturally on it own and many have salt added to enhance the flavor.

Adults should not eat more than about a teaspoon of salt in a day. If you have a health condition, it's better for you to eat less salt.

Stay away from fast food. It's not  only  high in fat, but it is also usually very high in salt.

**Cleanse your body by drinking enough water.**

 Drinking sufficient amount of water will assist your body flush out toxins, maintain your bodily functions, and keep your kidneys healthy. take at least eight 8-ounce glasses of water per day to stay hydrated, and take more if you are sweating, as a result of exercising or doing physical labor.

The amount of water  you need will be influenced by your body weight, your activity level, and the weather of your  environment.

 One of the best way to stay hydrated is to drink enough water that you don't feel thirsty.

If you urinate infrequently or pass dark or cloudy urine, you may need to drink more.

19

CHAPTER THREE

REDUCING STRESS.

**Protect your psychological well-being by maintaining close social relationships.**

Friends and family will make relaxation fun when things are taking good shapes and they can as well provide you with support and distraction when life is hard.

Maintain your social network through corresponding by writing, telephone, or in person. Using social media  also help people stay connected with friends and family.

Constant social interaction will help you relax and divert your mind off your stress.

If you feel isolated or bored, consider locating a support group or counselor to help you.

**Stay resilient by sleeping enough.**

By not getting a quality  sleep you are compounding the psychological stressors in your life with the physical stress of sleep deprivation.

While you sleep your body can put more energy into fighting against infections and healing.

 Try to have at least 7 to 8 hours of sleep per night. Some people may need even more because of individual differences.

**Stay excited about life through hobbies.**

This will give you reasons to be hopeful and prevent you from holding onto the things that are stressing you out.

Look for something that is not highly expensive which you can do all year long. Such as  reading, listening to music, art or photography, crafts, or sports

stop competitive activities that will subject you to additional pressure.

### Research illnesses.

 Spend some time to find out  on every illness on the NHS. This will enable  you to see every illness there is out there and you will also know what to avoid doing to stop you getting ill and if you do happen to get ill what your symptom/s could be. But this may take take time but it helps you a lot.

Take note of all the causes. When looking through all the illnesses take note of all the causes for everything. Try not to forget to note one down because you want to still do it. That does not favor your health one bit. For an example, some of the causes of meningitis is making use of toothbrushes, cigarettes others have used.

Take note of all the signs. Just like the causes, write down all the symptoms of all the illnesses as well. For example some symptoms of bacterial meningitis are a severe headache, fever, vomiting, drowsiness, confusion, seizures/fits, photophobia and a stiff neck. Also, note down the remedies if you notice these symptoms on yourself or your young child. For example, with meningitis, if you see these sign on anybody you must phone 999, or your local emergency service number as soon as possible.

Find out the test method for each illness. This will take long hours of studying, but learn a method to test if a person possibly has a certain illness off by heart.

**Consider becoming either vegan or vegetarian.**

 Research has shown that people who eat off of strict, healthy diets, such as vegan or vegetarian, live longer. Not eating of meat also reduces cholesterol and the risk of heart disease. If you choose one of these always take vitamin as supplement although vegan/vegetarian is fantastic for your body, you can be lacking some vitamins and some important nutrients. Take vitamins, you can even find vitamins specific for vegan/vegetarians at a Whole Foods or other health stores.

25

Ben Williams

www.ingramcontent.com/pod-product-compliance
Lightning Source LLC
Chambersburg PA
CBHW051429250726
48655CB00003B/1317